The

NATURAL REMEDIES

for

COMMON AILMENTS

Handbook

The
NATURAL REMEDIES
for
COMMON AILMENTS
Handbook

Celeste White, M.S.

Keswick House
Redding, CA

Copyright © 1996 Celeste White. Printed and bound in the United States of America. All rights reserved. No part of this book may be reproduced in any form or by any electronic or mechanical means including information storage and retrieval systems without permission in writing from the publisher, except by a reviewer, who may quote brief passages in a review. For information, please contact Keswick House, P O Box 992535, Redding, CA, 96099. First printing 1996.

The following names used in this volume are registered trademarks: Ace bandage, Boswellin Cream, Calming Essence, Celtic Sea Saltô, Earth Rite, Gripp-Heel, Metamucil, Mother Earth's, Q-tip, Scarmassage, Similasan, Traumeel, Rescue Remedy, Ziploc.

Although the author and publisher have extensively researched the material contained in this book to insure the accuracy of the information, we assume no responsibility for errors, inaccuracies, omissions, inconsistencies, or differences in individual responses to the remedies suggested. Any slights of people or organizations are unintentional. Readers should use their own judgment or consult their health care provider in applying specific treatments to their particular conditions.

Neither the publisher nor the author has any personal, financial, or business relationship to the companies mentioned in this book.

ISBN 0-9653024-0-7
Library of Congress Catalog No. 96-94470

First Edition
2 4 6 8 10 9 7 5 3 1

Cover design by Diane Morley and Candia Ludy

Additional copies are available. For your convenience, an order form is included in the back.

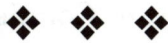

For the Otter

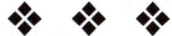

I would very much like to thank the following people for their input, feedback, expertise, and contributions:

Richard Hardie, M.Ed.
Aunt Connie
Frank Campanale, L.Ac.
Jack Kimple, M.D.
Joy Kimple, R.N., B.S., M.S.
Donald Sumers, L.Ac.
Patti Sumers
Patrick Moriarty
Kathleen Hardie, M.P.H.
Joseph Stenger, M.D.
Edwin Stewart, D.C.
Shadow Mountain Chiropractic
George Linville, M.S.W.
Ray Carlson, Ph.D.
Catherine White
Tim Schoch
Susannah Hardaway
Candia Ludy
Randy and Diane Manley
Mrs. Agard
Dean Patzman, D.D.S.

TABLE OF CONTENTS

Introduction i
Arthritis 2
Asthma and Allergies 4
Bruises and Sprains 8
Burns 10
Canker sores 12
Cold Sores/Fever blisters 12
Colds and Flu 14
Constipation 18
Cough 22
Cramps 24
Diarrhea 26
Eye Strain 28
Headaches 30
Hemorrhoids 34
Hiccups 36
Immune Function 38
Indigestion and Bloat 42

Itching:
: Insect bites and Poison oak/ivy 46

Scrapes and cuts 48

Sinus Problems 50

Stress and Depression 52

Appendix A:
: Phone numbers/addresses for manufacturers and distributors 56

Appendix B:
: The Natural Medicine Chest 58

Appendix C:
: Meditation technique 60

Appendix D:
: How to take homeopathic remedies 62

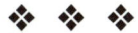

True Story

A woman went to her doctor complaining of headaches and dizziness. When the doctor entered the examining room, he asked his patient, "What seems to be the problem?" The woman told him, "It hurts and makes me dizzy when I do this." She proceeded to whip her head violently back and forth. Then she stopped. "What do you suggest?" she inquired. The doctor regarded her for a long time without speaking. Then he replied, "Don't do that."

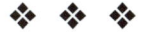

Introduction

This book is the result of twenty years' accumulation of information from many sources: herbalists, acupuncturists, allopathic healers, naturopaths, friends, family, folklore, books and studies. It contains remedies—some new, some timeworn—for most common ailments. I am also including the toll-free (usually) numbers and addresses of selected, reliable mail-order companies that carry homeopathic and herbal remedies. I have personally tried most of the remedies in this book and have chosen to include only those that have worked for me or for people I know.

Lots of over-the-counter remedies exist for many of these ailments, of course, and occasional use of these drugs is fine, in my opinion. I sometimes take ibuprofen for cramps, aspirin for a headache, or an antihistamine for allergies. However, regular use of these products poses several troublesome aspects:

1) Over-the-counter drugs add toxins to our already overloaded systems. 2) They have toxic, even lethal, overdoses. 3) Most have side-effects that weaken other parts of our systems and bodies. 4) Many lose their effectiveness over time. 5) They suppress symptoms rather than heal causes. 6) When we buy these products, we're funding an industry that is already mobilizing to limit or prevent our access to alternative and natural health care. 7) We're also paying for lots of annoying and negatively suggestive advertising.

But the most compelling reason for knowing about and using these remedies is their effectiveness. Some of the ones listed in this book are nothing short of amazing, and if medical science had come up with a drug that did the same thing, it would be the discovery of the century. Some of these remedies are subtle and work over time, but this is often the true route to healing. Not all of them work for everyone, however. Several possible treatments are usually presented for each ailment, so if one doesn't work for you, try another one.

Of course, serious conditions require a health care provider's supervision and care; but on a day-to-day basis, many of us just need to take care of simple health problems. And most of us want to do this without taking medication that can cause other health problems, dependency, or rebound effects. By learning to use natural home remedies, you can take care of your daily health safely and inexpensively; you can often prevent the development of serious conditions as well. And you can take the fate of your health out of the hands of profiteers and opportunists and put it back in your own.

Use these remedies wisely and enjoy good health!

❖ ❖ ❖
Natural Remedies
❖ ❖ ❖

ARTHRITIS

Regular exercise, a healthy diet that contains all necessary nutrients, and avoidance of processed and fast foods often helps keep arthritis at bay. However, if arthritis pain occurs, try the following:

- Rub cold-pressed peanut oil into the affected joints, particularly after bathing and before retiring. To keep your clothes and bedding from smelling like an old peanut, wrap oiled areas with strips of cloth or an ace bandage. Be sure to get unadulterated, cold-pressed peanut oil; The Heritage Store, which specializes in products formulated according to Edgar Cayce's diagnostic readings, sells a carefully prepared oil via mail order (See Appendix A for their toll free number).

- My 92-year-old Aunt Connie (who still throws dinner parties and is making plans to cruise up the Northwest Passage to Alaska) swears by a cream called Boswellin Cream, available through health food stores and made by a company called Nature's Herbs.

- BHI (Biologic Homeopathic Industries) makes a homeopathic arthritis tablet that many people find quite helpful (Check Appendix A for a mail order distributor).

- Drink lots of water. This can lead to marked improvement of symptoms.

- Acupuncture and acupressure are often quite effective in relieving arthritis.

- Stress can contribute to arthritis; develop a stress reduction program that works for you (See section on Stress).

- In recent tests, taking shark cartilage as a nutritional supplement before meals has proven to be highly effective over time.

- Take alfalfa tablets, three tablets four times a day, with meals.

- Teas (or herbal tablets or tinctures) made with the following herbs can provide relief, too: black cohosh, burdock, cayenne, Devil's claw, ginkgo, prickly ash, and sarsaparilla. Before mixing any of these herbs together, however, check with an herbalist to make sure that the combination is a safe one.

- Eat foods and drink juices made with cherries, ginger, and pineapple.

- Check with a kinesiologist, acupuncturist, or allergist to see if you have any food allergies, which can often contribute to arthritis.

❖ ❖ ❖

ASTHMA AND ALLERGIES

The incidence and lethality of asthma is on a dramatic rise, and many of us who suffer from asthma need to manage it under the supervision of a professional health care provider. This section includes many things that you can do to supplement your care, minimize your problems, and lessen your dependency on costly or toxic treatments. Given the environment that we live in, trying to follow all of these guidelines might prove difficult, if not impossible, so choose the ones that work for you and your lifestyle.

I have found that a combination of regular acupuncture treatments, herbal medicine, and chiropractic adjustments manage my asthma effectively, so that I rarely need to use an inhaler and I use antihistamines only a few weeks out of the year—quite a contrast to five years ago, when I was using a corticosteroid inhaler for both allergies and asthma, taking antihistamines six months out of the year, and asthma medication year round.

THINGS TO AVOID

- Artificial flavors, additives, food colorings, preservatives
- Tobacco smoke
- Aspirin, ibuprofen
- Animal dander
- Dust, which contains dust mites
- Partially hydrogenated oils
- Sugar, especially white sugar
- Foods that you are allergic to
- Alcohol, which can dehydrate your lungs and digestive tract; in particular, wine, which contains sulfites and tannins, can exacerbate asthma
- Perfumes and colognes, hair spray, heavily scented lotions and creams
- Fumes from paints and stains, solvents
- Hyperventilating; breathing from the top of your lungs
- Vigorous exercise in cold weather

THINGS TO TRY

- Keep your digestive system as healthy as possible; sluggish digestion can exacerbate asthma (see section on Constipation).

- Be sure to keep yourself hydrated; drink lots of pure, clean water.

- Use cold-pressed, unhydrogenated or monosaturated oils; in particular, use olive oil, which will also keep your cholesterol levels down.

- Several companies sell homeopathic asthma tablets, for regular use or when an asthma attack strikes. BHI makes a good asthma tablet, which is carried by mail order distributor Shanah Azee. In addition, a company called BioEngergetics makes extremely effective homeopathic allergy drops (See Appendix A).

- Visualization and relaxation techniques are quite helpful; imagine your bronchioles as relaxed and well-dilated.

- Eat a teaspoon or two of local honey daily.

- Wash new clothes before wearing them; most are sprayed with formaldehyde, which can trigger asthma.

- Thoroughly air out any clothing or bedding that has been dry cleaned.

- Use natural cleaning products in your home. Earth Rite makes good products for a variety of uses. THE NONTOXIC HOME AND OFFICE, by Debra Lynn Dadd, gives ingredients and directions for making your own cleaning products.

- Use natural products when building or remodeling your home: wood, tile, wool carpet (though some people have an allergy to wool and should use something else), metal.

- Acupressure points often work for me in a pinch, too. Count down three ribs from your collar bone and dig your index fingers into the little socket formed between the ribs (both above and below your third rib; do one set, then the next) and against the breast bone where the ribs attach. Apply pressure for several minutes.

    Another set of points that often works is located about an inch or so below your collar bone. Find it by clasping the tendon that leads from your arm to your chest. Your fingers will be tucked into your armpit and your thumbs should be resting on the acupressure spot. Poke around a little bit to find a sore place; if you discover one, dig your thumbs in there, or use your fingers. Apply pressure for several minutes.

❖ ❖ ❖

BRUISES AND SPRAINS

If there is a possibility you've broken a bone, you should get X-rays. But if all that's happened is something like, say . . . your partner dropped the balpeen hammer on your toe while you two were trying to get the VCR to work—and you're certain that all you have is a bad bruise or a sprain—try these steps:

- For a bruise, rub the area vigorously for several minutes, even though it will hurt.

- Then apply the magical, amazing Traumeel cream, made by the German company, Heel; it prevents swelling, discoloration, and pain. One of the major active ingredients is *Arnica*, but it also contains a whole host of other wonderful healing herbs. Traumeel is often available at your local health food store, or you can order it from Shanah Azee (see Appendix A). Put it on as soon as possible and keep applying it as necessary.

- Apply ice or a cold compress to either a bad bruise or a sprain. Twenty minutes is usually plenty.

- Immobilize a sprain. Wrap it firmly with an Ace bandage or adhesive tape to restrict unnecessary movement, but be sure not to wrap it too tightly. You don't want to cut off all your circulation. Elevating an injured limb for awhile helps, too, as does keeping use of the limb or digit in question to a minimum.

- Oral Traumeel tablets are also quite helpful and are available from Shanah Azee (Appendix A). As a matter of fact, I fractured my kneecap once in a bike accident, and with the combination of Traumeel ointment and tablets, I didn't even need to take any pain meds.

- If you hit a blood vessel or an artery, you can sometimes end up with a hematoma, which is a lump formed under the skin from pooled blood that then coagulates. Gently rub the area until the lump disappears; use hot soaks, too.

BURNS

A burn can leave an ugly scar and pose a risk of infection, too, if not dealt with properly. In fact, however, unless a large portion of skin is badly burned, you can easily heal a nasty burn scar- and infection-free. One of the best things you can do is to keep an *Aloe vera* plant growing in your kitchen or someplace in your house. These plants are as miraculous for burns as Traumeel ointment is for bruises and sprains. The active ingredients are very fragile, however, so buying *Aloe vera* lotion, concentrate, or gel is not the same thing at all as having a fresh, living plant at your disposal. Fortunately, they are hardy and forgiving and will grow under the most thankless, tenuous conditions.

- As soon as possible, run cold water over the burn for several minutes. DO NOT apply ice.

- Cut off a portion of an *Aloe vera* leaf, split it lengthwise with a knife (trimming off the little spikes on the side if you want, to avoid scratching yourself—and it's not a bad idea to thank the plant for its contribution), and smear the goo all over the burn. Reapply whenever the burn starts to ache. The goo tastes extremely bitter, so remember this if you're putting it near your mouth or on your hands.

- *Aloe vera* also works great for bad sunburns. Just cut the leaves as described and smear them all over yourself.

- Once the burn starts to heal, apply calendula ointment (obtainable from BHI; see Appendix A) or vitamin E oil.

- If you do end up with a scar, Scarmassage ointment, which is available from Heritage products (a mail order company that specializes in Edgar Cayce remedies; see Appendix A for their toll-free number), is very effective over time in reducing or erasing scars. I prefer the liquid roll-on; you just apply it to the scar twice a day for several months. If you're persistent, I think you'll be quite pleased with the results.

❖ ❖ ❖

CANKER SORES

Stress and an over-acidic constitution caused by eating too many sweets or processed foods can predispose us to canker sores. Avoiding these things can often keep them from appearing. If you get one, however, the most effective strategy I've discovered—which really works! —is to apply alum powder to the canker sore. Scoop up a little on your finger and then dab it on. It stings like crazy, but it cauterizes the wound, which can then start to heal. Alum is used in pickling and can usually be found in the spice section of the grocery store.

COLD SORES/FEVER BLISTERS

Again, fever blisters (also called cold sores) are highly stress related, so the less stress you experience, the less likely you are to get one of these unpleasant little buggers. However, when fever blisters rear their ugly head, I have found two very effective ways of dealing with them, one a preventative, one that hastens their disappearance.

- Most people who suffer from fever blisters on their face know when they are about to erupt; the skin turns red and tingles. If this happens, rub pure vitamin E oil on that patch of skin (you can even puncture a vitamin E capsule and smear the liquid on). Apply it liberally. The majority of the time, one application is enough, but you can keep an eye on the trouble spot and apply the vitamin E as often as you feel necessary. Usually, the fever blister never appears after this.

- If the cold sore occurs anyway, soften the scab with a little warm water on a wash cloth (be sure no one else uses the cloth and that you wash it before using it for anything else). Then crush a vitamin C tablet in a cup or bowl and mix up a little slurry with a few mls. of warm water. Using a Q-tip, swab the slurry on the fever blister several times a day. This, too, will sting, but it will also cause the fever blister to clear up much faster and often soothes the constant ache. Powdered vitamin C is also available from the Heritage Store (see Appendix A) and can be used in place of a crushed tablet.

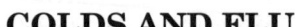

COLDS AND FLU

Colds and flu have become rather epidemic lately, another side-effect of our high-stress lives and highly challenged immune systems. Even if we're in good health, we're often surrounded by people who aren't. The following steps can help you either to avoid coming down with these ailments entirely, or they can make the duration much less miserable:

- *Echinacea* is a widely used herb these days, but finding good quality is difficult. *Echinacea* has several different constituents, some of them water soluble, some of them alcohol soluble. The *Echinacea* you use should have both in order to be truly effective. Again, the fresher the herb, the better. The Herb Pharm in Oregon makes an excellent tincture (see Appendix A). Mix the recommended number of drops in a little bit of water and drink, three or four times a day; more frequently if it feels like you're really coming down with something vile. You can tell good, potent *Echinacea* by the puckery little tingle it gives you a few delayed seconds or minutes after drinking it. I wouldn't recommend taking it straight.

- Zinc has also been shown to reduce the severity of a cold. Zinc lozenges can be obtained at your local health food store. Suck them slowly, rather than crunching them down the way I'm always tempted to do.

- The German homeopathic company, Heel, makes a wonderful cold and flu remedy called Gripp-Heel (available from Shanah Azee mail order; see Appendix A for their toll free number). At the first signs of a cold or flu, dissolve one tablet under your tongue four times a day.

- A former chiropractor of mine swears by the following preventative (and she was the only one who didn't come down with the lingering, hacking, creeping crud that decimated Colorado that summer): Take three alfalfa tablets four times a day, preferably with meals.

- Eat plenty of garlic, both fresh and cooked. Different properties are present in the different preparations. One good way to get fresh garlic into your diet is to squeeze copious amounts into salad dressings. Claim that you then have to stay home from work, to spare your fellow employees.

- Eat freshly prepared chicken soup made from scratch. There really is something fabulous in there, though modern science can't figure out what yet.

- Guzzle fluids, preferably water or freshly squeezed fruit and vegetable juices. Avoid sugary drinks or diet drinks.

- Of course, many people find taking large doses of vitamin C to be helpful, anywhere from 2000 to 5000 mg. a day.

- Cut back on all sugar intake.

- Better-tasting and way more fun than any over-the-counter nighttime cold and flu remedies is a brew recommended by an Irish friend of ours: Make a hot toddy by placing a heaping tsp. of honey, three or four whole cloves, and an ounce or two of whiskey in the bottom of a mug. Fill the cup with boiling water and drink it as hot as you can stand. This will help you to sweat out some toxins and provide a delightfully relaxed, drowsy feeling before going to bed.

- For a sore throat, gargle several times a day with warm to hot salt water (about a quarter tsp. salt per half cup water). This is extremely effective, especially if you jump right on it.

- Many herbalists recommend taking the herb *Lomatium*. You might be able to find it at your local health food store, or you can order a tincture through Shanah Azee mail order (check out Appendix A). Beware that some people are sensitive to this herb, however, and that this can cause a rash, as can taking too large a dosage. More is not better.

- Rent comedies and watch them on your VCR. Or pick up books by authors you think are funny and read them. If you have a frustrated comedian for a friend or a silly spouse or family member, ask them to entertain you in person or by phone for a few minutes. A good laugh will boost your immune system and helps to clear your lungs.

- One thing that you should NOT do is take antibiotics for a cold or flu. Antibiotics are effective only against bacterial infections, not viruses, and their effectiveness against bacteria has been compromised because of over-prescription and indiscriminate use. If a sinus or respiratory infection hangs on and on, check with your physician; you may have a bacterial infection, in which case antibiotics might be appropriate. These days, some people even prefer to avoid antibiotics for bacterial infections; they treat them instead with herbs and/or homeopathics prescribed by their health care provider.

- Let yourself be sick occasionally and rest. Don't put pressure on yourself to leap up the minute you feel the tiniest bit better and start putting together advertising campaigns, theses, or school plays.

❖ ❖ ❖

CONSTIPATION

Yuk. Constipation. Anyone who's ever experienced it knows how unpleasant it can be. Long term constipation can also increase your risk of colon cancer and other diseases. For some people, adding bran to their diet or taking psyllium seed (in the form of Metamucil or some other brand) is enough to keep them regular. Some of us, however, need to be more diligent and creative, especially women right before their periods. The following remedies have proven extremely useful for me and countless others:

- It's always a good idea to include lots of fresh fruits and leafy vegetables in your diet. A minimum of two pieces of fruit and a big salad or plate of steamed vegetables a day is not a bad goal.

- I also find that the timing of when I eat certain foods helps as much as the food item itself. Eating an apple or pear right before I go to bed has proved extremely effective.

- Take four to six alfalfa tablets with a glass of water just before retiring.

- Be sure to drink lots and lots of water. This alone can sometimes help.

- Include bran and high fiber foods in your diet. I bought one of those cool bread-making machines, and I add oat or wheat bran to all the whole grain loaves I make.

- Once every couple of months, engage in an intestinal cleanse. Purchase high grade psyllium seed from your local health food store (Sonne's and Veico are good brands) and the accompanying herb tablets that contain *Cascara sagrada* and *Aloe curcao*. The first night, take two herb tablets along with a tumbler full of water and a heaping teaspoon of the psyllium seed. I sweeten the water with about a quarter cup of apple juice or cranberry juice. Be sure to stir up the psyllium seed immediately and frantically upon adding it to the liquid in the tumbler. Then drink it as fast as you can. Otherwise, you might end up with a glass of solid gel, fit only for punk hairdo styling. The next two nights, take just one herb tablet along with a glass of water and heaping tsp. of psyllium seed.

- Many people also find that caffeine in the form of coffee or black tea acts as a laxative. For some people, however, caffeine can have exactly the opposite effect; so if you're experiencing persistent, stubborn constipation, you might try giving up caffeine for awhile and see if that helps. (Warning: Cold turkeying off caffeine can cause headaches.)

- Avoid eating too much dairy, red meat, sugar, chocolate, and processed foods.

- For some people, hot, spicy foods help keep things moving, as does plenty of garlic in the diet. Try adding fresh ginger to your diet, too; ginger promotes healthy elimination.

- Getting plenty of exercise is important.

- Before you go to sleep and when you wake up, massage your abdomen. Seek out any spots that seem to contain lumpy blockages and rub them gently but firmly (if you experience any pain, contact your doctor). Finish by rubbing your tummy in a clockwise spiral, starting at your bellybutton and widening your circle with each stroke. Do this several times.

- Another practice that helps quite a bit is to breathe from your diaphragm and abdomen, rather than from your chest. The movement of food through our digestive system works by peristaltis, a sort of squeezing, rippling motion of the intestines; so when we breathe properly, this adds to the activity of these organs and moves things along more speedily.

"*Health is a state of complete physical, mental, and social well-being and not merely the absence of disease or infirmity...*"

—*Constitution of the World Health Organization, July 22, 1946*

COUGH

I once had a cough that I thought I would never get rid of. It lasted for months. And it was a terrible, wracking, convulsive sort of a thing, the kind of cough where people back away from you nervously, dogs bark at you, and public health officials start moving in for a quarantine. I thought at one point that I'd cracked a rib from coughing. If only I knew about the following remedies *then*!

- The homeopathic company BHI makes a cough tablet that is truly miraculous. When my husband used to get a cough, it would keep him up all night. No more! Not only that, we once had a friend come visit who had a killer cough, which, he said, nothing had come close to touching. We gave him one of these tablets, and he never coughed again! It was kind of spooky. Check out Appendix A for a distributor.

- The Heritage Store (the Edgar Cayce people) also makes a wonderful cough syrup and respiratory tonic called Mother Earth's. It not only soothes your cough, it strengthens your pulmonary system. (See Appendix A for their toll-free number.)

- If you have neither of these remedies on hand and you need something quick, make a nice old-fashioned and very effective cough syrup from whiskey, honey, and lemon juice. For a single dose, squeeze a quarter of a fresh lemon and mix the juice with a scant teaspoon of honey and a teaspoon of whiskey.

CRAMPS

Cramps can make you absolutely miserable. They can make it difficult to do or concentrate on anything else. Mild exercise such as walking often helps, even though all you might feel like doing is writhing on the bed or floor. Meditation or relaxation techniques can also help. In addition, try the following:

- Take 800 I.U. units of vitamin E a day, for several days before and during your period.

- The following method can be a little messy and it involves some paraphernalia, but it can be very effective. Find an old hand towel or piece of flannel that you don't plan on using for anything else. Buy high quality castor oil (The Heritage Store carries some; see Appendix A) and put some into a squeeze bottle. Lying on your bed or on the floor, place the flannel on your abdomen and drench it with the oil (but not so much that you drizzle it all over your bed or floor; on second thought, you might want to have a towel underneath you, too). Then cover that with another old bath towel that you're not particularly fond of, then lay a warm heating pad on top of that. Leave it on for thirty minutes or so. Afterwards, you can swab the oil off with witch hazel or alcohol. I keep my old flannel and towel in a plastic bag for future use.

- Certain yoga postures can also ease cramping. These days, just about every town boasts at least one yoga instructor; call around to find a good class. One nice side benefit of taking yoga, too, is that it will improve your overall health and flexibility.

- If all else fails, take some ibuprofen.

- For PMS sufferers, try PMS Relief, homeopathic drops made by BioEnergetics (see Appendix A for their toll-free number).

DIARRHEA

Diarrhea is often caused by a bacterium or virus, in which case, it's best to just let things run their course. I'll never forget the time I was heading off to Nova Scotia on a camping trip, and I decided to take some medication that would stop the diarrhea I had developed a few days before. Ba-a-ad idea. Halfway up the coast, I developed viral encephalitis; I ended up with a headache that made me beg my husband to shoot me, to put me out of my misery. For awhile, I thought I had a brain tumor, I slept through the entire vacation, and instead of eating all the yummy fresh fish and new potatoes that were plentiful everywhere, all I could stomach was chicken noodle soup. It was a drag. I really think that if I'd just let my body get rid of what it wanted to, I wouldn't have become so sick. If you suffer from diarrhea on a chronic basis, however, you should consult a health care provider. For occasional or mild problems, try the following remedies:

- Eat foods high in starch like bread, potatoes, and pasta.

- Stress can be a major cause of diarrhea. If this is your problem, work on coming up with a relaxation program, as ignoring this symptom can inflict long term damage to your digestive system.

- Some foods cause diarrhea, particularly milk, if you are lactose intolerant. Try drinking milk that has acidophilus added to it or use milk substitutes (be sure to get plenty of calcium from other sources). Other problem foods include: acidic fruits, high fiber fruits and vegetables, foods high in fat, alcohol, and caffeine.

- Bananas are often good for ameliorating diarrhea (Hmm, that last phrase has sort of a ring to it, doesn't it? Sounds like a Victorian novel for young ladies.) Other fruits high in pectin, such as apples, plums, cranberries, red currants, quinces and gooseberries, can be helpful, too.

- Taking antibiotics can cause diarrhea because they kill the bacteria in your digestive system. To repopulate your intestinal flora, eat yogurt with live cultures, drink acidophilus milk, or take acidophilus culture in powder form.

❖ ❖ ❖

EYE STRAIN

Eye strain is a real problem these days, especially with all the computer use. When you're reading or working on a computer, be sure to blink a lot and to vary your focal length. Take a break often and stare out the window or let your gaze travel around the room, resting on different objects. It's also a good idea to let your eyes go out of focus every now and then, to give them a rest.

- Try eye exercises, at least once a day. One exercise is to hold your index finger up in front of your face, focus on it, then move your finger away from and toward your face. Do this several times.

    Another exercise is to roll your eyes up as high as they will go in their sockets (without straining) and then to gradually start moving them back and forth in ever-widening arcs, sort of like a pendulum, until you're rolling them from one corner of your eye, all the way to the top of your socket, to the other corner.

    Still another exercise is to squeeze your eyes shut as tightly as you can and hold this position for a few seconds.

    (Caution: To avoid looking silly to others, do these exercises in private only.)

- BHI makes a homeopathic eye tablet that is often helpful.

- Placing freshly cut cucumber slices on your closed eyes is soothing and relaxing.

- You can also try filling a pint-sized Ziploc bag with cool water from your tap, lying down and placing the bag on your eyes.

- Similasan, a Swiss company, makes a very nice herbal eye drop. You can get these drops at your local health food store, or from Home Health mail order distributors (see Appendix A for their toll-free number).

- Some people find that taking the herb Eyebright is very beneficial. The Heritage Store carries a nice product in gel caps (see Appendix A).

HEADACHE

There are lots of reasons for headaches, so if you're having them on a frequent basis, you should see your health care practitioner. Causes can range from allergies to stress to viral infections to eye strain. Well, okay, brain tumors, too, but fortunately, they are very rare. Odds are, your headache is not caused by a brain tumor, but entertaining the possibility is always good for an adrenalin jolt. For an occasional headache, the use of over-the-counter pain killers isn't a bad thing, but chronic use not only adds drugs and toxins to your system, you would be better off identifying the root cause and clearing up the problem. Check the following suggestions and see if any of them apply to your situation.

- Drink a couple of glasses of water right away and keep yourself hydrated. Headaches are often caused by dehydration, especially after exercising, sitting in a hot tub or sauna, or working so hard that you forget to keep yourself hydrated. Avoid alcohol and sugared drinks, as these will only worsen the problem.

- Given up caffeinated drinks lately? This could give you headaches. Try weaning yourself off coffee or black tea slowly, rather than stopping all at once.

- If your headaches are associated with other allergy symptoms, you might have a sinus headache. Try BioEnergetics' homeopathic allergy and/or sinus drops. Several Chinese herb combinations also help for allergies and sinuses, too; so if these drops don't clear up your headaches, try a good acupuncturist/Chinese herbalist.

- Sinus problems in general can give you a headache. See section on Sinus Infections.

- Eye strain, too, can cause headaches. See section on Eye Strain. If problems persist, get your vision checked; you may need glasses.

- Exposure to certain fumes and chemicals such as gasoline, dry cleaning solvents, pesticides, household cleaners, tobacco smoke, copy machine toner, and even perfumes and colognes can give you headaches. Try to avoid these substances whenever possible, using natural substitutes when available (Check out the book, THE NONTOXIC HOME AND OFFICE, by Debra Lynn Dadd). When working with volatile or toxic chemicals, always make sure that your work area is well-ventilated. Work outside if possible, or consider renting a respirator type mask to work in. Dust masks will not screen out volatile chemicals.

- Stress and tension headaches can be relieved by meditation or relaxation techniques (see Appendix C).

- Massage your face and head with your fingers and thumbs. Find any sore or tender places and concentrate on them. One area that often needs attention is the two spots right underneath your eyebrows on either side of the bridge of your nose. Try a little acupressure or massage on these two spots, using your thumbs or knuckles. Other problem areas include the temples, the spots right above your ears, a band across the middle of your forehead, and the places on the back of your skull where it attaches to your neck.

- If your headache is caused by a cold, flu, or other virus, you may just need to take a couple of aspirin and go to bed.

"Human beings represent the juncture between Heaven and Earth, the offspring of their union, a fusion of cosmic and terrestrial forces."

—*H. Beinfield and E. Korngold;*
BETWEEN HEAVEN AND EARTH

HEMORRHOIDS

I think hemorrhoids are one of those plagues the cosmos decided to visit upon mankind in order to keep us humble. Not only are they painful, they're embarrassing! Nobody wants to admit to having them, except for the highly paid actors and actresses on television advertisements. And then you wonder, how do they feel when that commercial comes flashing on the screen and they're sitting there watching "Unsolved Mysteries" with all of their friends? At any rate, hemorrhoids are preventable and treatable. Try the following remedies:

- Keep your digestive system healthy and regular. Most hemorrhoids are formed from straining. See the section on Constipation.

- Swab the area several times a day with a cotton ball soaked in witch hazel. This is a lot cheaper than buying commercially prepared wipes.

- Apply calendula ointment (see Appendix A for a source) and/or vitamin E oil.

- If you have a hemorrhoid, this is one of the few times that playing with something is okay. A hemorrhoid is pooled, coagulated blood that needs to get redissolved into the bloodstream.

When you're in the shower or bath, fiddle around with the little bugger—rub it, massage it, stroke it. If you find yourself enjoying this, don't feel guilty; just don't tell anybody about it. Except maybe your closest friends. Maybe.

- Warm or hot soaks, either in the tub or in a sitz bath or using a washcloth, are good, too. This also helps to redissolve the coagulated blood.

HICCUPS

Some people don't get hiccups, like my husband, but I get them fairly frequently and they drive me nuts! Putting a paper bag over my head never worked, scaring me never worked—though it's always a kick when people go to the trouble to work out something elaborate and sneaky enough to scare me—eating a spoonful of sugar never worked. However, the following remedies have proven quite effective:

- Take your index finger and press right on the base of that flap of cartilage that leads to your ear canal, above your earlobe and adjacent to your cheekbone. In fact, nuzzle your finger into the socket formed by your cheekbone and your jaw, but make sure you're still pushing up against your ear. While pressing firmly on this spot, take a tiny little sip of water. For some reason, a tiny little sip is more effective than a big gulp.

- Drink nine swallows of water in succession, without taking a breath in between. Nine seems to be the magic number, though I can't explain why.

- If you're not hiccuping so hard that this is impossible, try breathing from your diaphragm as deeply, evenly, and rhythmically as you can.

- While standing up, take a few gulps of water from the opposite side of the glass. This is by far the most awkward of the hiccup remedies, but it is an excellent test of one's coordination, and it's always good for a few laughs.

- Some people find that by taking their thumbs and pressing into the back of their heads where the muscles attach from their necks, they can stop their hiccups. Sometimes it's easier if you can get someone else to do this for you.

❖ ❖ ❖

IMMUNE FUNCTION

These days, our immune systems are under an almost continual assault: from chemicals in our food, water, air, and buildings, a highly disruptive electromagnetic environment, over-crowding, traffic, economic woes, dysfunctional families, crime, stressful employment situations, emerging new diseases, and too much to do in too little time. Coping well with stress is one of the most important things we can do to strengthen our immune system (see section on Stress and Depression), but there are some other tricks to employ, too:

- Regular acupuncture or acupressure can help avert illness before it develops. Because these methods work on balancing our overall system and address energy blockages before they become organic problems, they represent the best preventative medicine we have available, in my opinion.

- Be sure to get plenty of rest. Despite what some people think, sleeping is not a waste of time; our bodies use sleep to make repairs, process necessary information, maintain healthy perception, and to heal.

- *Echinacea* also boosts our immune system. See the section on Colds and Flu to get more information on this wonderful herb. Be sure to obtain *Echinacea* that contains all the active components, some of which are water soluble, others of which are alcohol soluble.

- *Astralagus* is another herb that has been shown to improve immune function. It's available in tablets as a nutritional supplement. Your local health food store, as well as other reliable herb suppliers, will likely have it in stock.

- Keeping your electromagnetic field in balance can also give a boost to your immune system. Avoid placing beds against a wall that rests against the back of a television in another room. The wavelengths produced by the television go right through the wall and are the strongest from the back of the set. Similarly, don't place a bed near the spot where the electrical box to your house is located. Keep exposure to all electromagnetic fields to a minimum. For example, use a hand razor instead of an electric one, rake instead of using a leaf blower. Use an electromagnetic screen on your computer and don't sit or sleep closer than four feet to either side or the back of the computer when it's on.

  In addition, a pocket diode that keeps your energy field in balance can be purchased from The Heritage Store (See Appendix A).

- Several studies have shown that individuals' moods and attitudes have a direct, biochemical bearing on the strength of their immune systems. Emotions often get short shrift in this society, but you will be healthier if you deal with any emotional or relationship problems you might have and don't put this off. If you need counseling or therapy, get it. Express your feelings. Laugh a lot. Cry when you need to. Forgive people, including yourself.

  Check out flower remedies, first developed by Dr. Bach, an English physician, which address different emotional difficulties (See Appendix A for sources; see section on Stress for a bit more discussion).

"I can't imagine anybody thinking that the mind and the body could be separate in view of the multiplicity of connections from the brain to virtually all systems."

—David Felton, M.D., Ph.D., from
HEALING AND THE MIND,
by Bill Moyers

INDIGESTION AND BLOAT

Often, we get indigestion because we make pigs of ourselves. When we eat too much, our digestive system gets overloaded and can't effectively process the food. If we gobble our food, too, that causes problems, as does eating when we're stressed out. Stress creates excess stomach acid which leads to stomach upset. So, if we eat smaller portions, dine in a leisurely fashion (to give our brains time to catch up with our stomachs and realize we're actually full), and truly focus on and enjoy the whole gastronomic experience, we will have fewer problems with indigestion. In addition, try these remedies:

- Indigestion can be caused by eating foods that don't agree with us. Keep a diary to see if there is any particular food or foods that give you indigestion. Some people have borderline allergies to things such as nuts, seafood, strawberries, wheat, dairy, etc. I find that raw onions and broccoli (honest!) don't agree with me; spicy foods also give some people trouble. Eliminating these items from your diet can help a great deal.

- Avoid eating too much fat. For some people, this can send their gall bladder into shock, shipping too much bile into their intestines, with resulting stomach pain and upset.

- Milk is a problem for people who have lactose intolerance. However, before giving up on milk entirely—if you like it—try drinking milk that has acidophilus added to it. Pasteurization kills the bacteria and denatures the enzymes that makes milk easily digestible. Raw milk is also more digestible because it hasn't been pasteurized, but some people feel nervous about the idea of drinking milk that hasn't been treated. I've drunk raw milk for years, however, with no problems.

- You can also take acidophilus in powdered form. It's available at your local health food stores; some grocery stores carry it, too. Add it to a glass of water and drink, three times a day, or once at night before you go to bed.

- Fennel, coriander seed, fenugreek, licorice, and ginger all help digestion. Adding these to your diet can be quite helpful. In fact, that little mixture that you often find at the cash register as you leave Indian restaurants is a wonderful digestive aid—you know, that combination of toasted fennel seeds, coriander seeds, licorice bits, etc. If you can find some, keep it on hand for a post-prandial treat. Or buy the ingredients, toast the seeds, and mix up your own.

- Another tactic that works for some people, though it can be a hassle to pull this off, is to avoid eating starches and proteins at the same time. Most fruits and vegetables can be eaten with either one (though acidic fruits and starches aren't the best match).

- Drinking too much water with your meals can dilute stomach acid and make it difficult to digest your food properly. Drink water sparingly during meals; drink it copiously in between meals.

- Drinking wine with meals, especially rich or fatty ones, can often serve as a digestive aid. Drinking red wine will also keep your cholesterol levels down. The French tend to eat a fairly high fat diet, but their cholesterol levels are lower than Americans'. Several researchers feel that drinking wine with meals, particularly red wine, makes the difference. Of course, don't overdo it.

- Now, this might sound suspicious or fishy or bogus, but I find, in fact, that often a small portion of a sweet after a big meal helps to finish things off in a most satisfying, well-balanced way. Don't gorge, of course, because this will just make things worse. Just try indulging in a nice, little tasty dessert.

- Often, a cola drink is just the thing to settle your stomach. Both Home Health and Heritage Store sell a natural cola syrup to make up your own beverage (Appendix A).

- Mint is an excellent digestive aid. Eat a mint after dinner, or brew yourself a cup of peppermint or spearmint tea. People who suffer from esophogeal reflux (AKA heartburn) might want to avoid mint after meals, though, as it tends to relax the stomach sphincter.

- Sometimes eating too much fiber, particularly all at one time, can cause bloating and gas. If you're starting a new fiber-rich diet, try cutting back until you find a comfortable compromise.

- Vitamin B-6 has been shown to reduce bloating in women who suffer from PMS. By far the best source of B vitamins comes from nutritional yeast. Nutritional yeast, a flaky, yellow powder, can be found at health food stores, often in bulk. The good thing about nutritional yeast, as opposed to supplements, is that it provides all the B vitamins in the most beneficial, effective ratios, as nature intended. I mix up a couple of heaping teaspoonfuls in a glass of vegetable juice and drink it once a day. Another way to use nutritional yeast (which, by the way, is yummier by far than Brewer's yeast) is to sprinkle it, along with dill and a little salt, on popcorn. This gives the popcorn a tasty, cheeselike flavor.

- Of course, there's the tried and true bicarbonate of soda remedy. Mix a half teaspoon of baking soda in 4 oz. of water and drink.

❖ ❖ ❖

ITCHING
INSECT BITES AND POISON OAK, IVY

Fortunately, I now live in an area that does not contain CHIGGERS, the worst itching nemesis I know of, but we still get plenty of bug bites and we have poison oak all over the place. We also have some fairly creepy, Twilight Zone insects like cone-nosed beetles that crawl onto you, insert their disgusting little proboscis into your skin and feed for twenty minutes or so while you're sleeping. It's gross! But for some people, insect stings and bites of creatures like the cone-nosed beetle are worse than gross, they can cause severe anaphylactic reactions. These individuals should keep an emergency insect sting kit handy. And these days, any ticks you find on yourself you should keep in a little vial or jar for possible identification of Lyme's disease, should you find yourself developing any symptoms (especially fever, joint pain, and the characteristic bull's eye rash around the tick bite). Otherwise, try these remedies for less drastic situations:

- If you've been exposed to poison oak or ivy, wash the area/s with cool water and soap.

- My cousin, who had been suffering from poison oak rashes quite a bit, swears by this homeopathic remedy: Poison Oak/Poison Ivy Relief, made by Natra-Bio out of Ferndale, WA, available through your local health food store.

- For most mosquito and flea bites, etc., I find swabbing the bite with witch hazel and then rubbing calendula ointment on it to provide wonderful relief.

- If you live in chigger country, this is what we used to do when I was a kid: It's not exactly natural, but we would dab a little clear nail polish on the bite, which would suffocate the chigger. Then the bite would clear up and the itching would cease a lot faster.

- For insect stings, flick any remaining stinger out with your fingernail, then make a paste out of water and baking soda and pack it on the sting.

- For ticks, pinch their bodies as close to your skin as possible and pluck them out; twisting is no longer recommended. Be sure to clean the bite with alcohol or hydrogen peroxide. Also, save the infernal insect in the aforementioned vial or jar until you're sure you have no symptoms of Lyme's disease. Or, line them up in a little display on your mantel for a nifty conversation piece.

❖ ❖ ❖

SCRAPES AND CUTS

Probably most people know what to do about a cut or scrape: wash thoroughly with soap and water, flush with hydrogen peroxide and then cover with a bandage. Sometimes it's a good idea to smear a little antibiotic cream on the bandage, but it's also a good idea to keep antibiotic use to a minimum. Currently, a large number of bacteria are developing resistance, in very short time periods, to all kinds of antibiotics. Recent research suggests that bacteria are able to evolve "intelligently," to acquire resistance to antibiotics in their environment faster than would be expected from mutation and natural selection alone. Personally, I think we need to try to develop a different relationship to microorganisms: Rather than try to wipe them all out, which would be extremely biologically destructive (we wouldn't be able to digest our food without the bacteria in our intestines, for example), we need to strengthen our immune systems, as well as improve our understanding of their ecology and relationship to their hosts (i.e., us).

- If you find microorganisms invading your wound to the point that it becomes infected, one of the most effective things to do is to soak it several times a day in hot salt water. This draws out the infection and helps to sterilize it as well.

- Keep the wound aerated, too. Leave the bandage off when there is no longer bleeding or a risk that dirt will get into the wound. Scrapes are more likely to get infected than cuts are, so be sure to clean scrapes thoroughly, even debriding the area if necessary, and giving them plenty of exposure to the air.

- For nasty cuts that aren't quite bad enough for stitches, use butterfly strips to close the wound.

- If the wound leaves a scar, apply Scarmassage liquid or cream, a highly effective Edgar Cayce formula (See Appendix A, The Heritage Store, for a supplier).

❖ ❖ ❖

SINUS PROBLEMS

Sinus problems have several different causes: allergies, colds and flu, and sinus infections. They can give you splitting headaches and make you feel like your entire brain cavity is filled with mucus. I'll never forget the sinus infection I got in college; when it began to clear up and I started blowing my nose, I honestly thought my head was going to cave in before it was all over. Whatever the cause, I've found the following remedies to be wonderfully effective for sinus congestion.

- Try BioEnergetics homeopathic Sinus Drops (See Appendix A). We have a friend who was taking over-the-counter sinus medication every day for years. This wasn't too kind to his liver, but it kept him from getting blinding, incapacitating headaches. The first time he tried these sinus drops, he got a nosebleed, but then afterwards, his sinuses and headaches cleared up to an amazing degree. He takes his former medication only a couple of times a month now.

- That excellent homeopathic company, Heel, makes an herbal nasal spray that has no rebound effects and is quite effective. It's called Euphorbium Nasal Spray and it can be obtained through Shanah Azee (Appendix A).

- This method was recommended to me by my acupuncturist: First, obtain some good salt (Celtic sea salt is the best, or any other kind of salt that isn't all dried out when you buy it; try your local health food store or write to The Grain & Salt Society in Appendix A for their fine product, Celtic Sea Saltô). Have on hand hydrogen peroxide, a dropper, mortar and pestle, and one of those rubber bulbs that people use to irrigate kids' ears with. You know the kind—they look sort of like a miniature dark blue gourd with a skinny neck. Take a pinch of salt and grind it up with a mortar and pestle. Then add a few ounces of water, enough so that the resultant mixture tastes like seawater (you don't want it too concentrated or this will dry out your sinuses). Add 5 to 10 drops of hydrogen peroxide to the mixture with the dropper, stir it all up, then draw up some of the liquid in the rubber bulb. Tipping your head back a bit, put the rubber bulb to one of your nostrils and squeeze, not too hard. Saltwater will go rushing into your sinus cavities and dribbling down the back of your throat and running down the front of your face, so have some tissue or a towel handy. Then repeat for the other nostril. Do it a couple more times, then blow your nose. It's not really very pleasant, but the end result can be truly refreshing and cleansing.

❖ ❖ ❖

STRESS AND DEPRESSION

I've put these two together because I believe they go hand in hand. Depression does have a genetic, biochemical component to it, but I think that the triggers are emotional and stress-related. Coping well with stress often means avoiding or alleviating depression. Handling stress in a constructive, effective manner also helps to prevent or clear up other ailments such as stress-related headaches, ulcers and colitis, skin rashes, anxiety, insomnia, asthma, and perhaps even cancer, heart disease, and autoimmune disorders. Keeping stress in our environment to a minimum is desirable, of course, and should certainly be pursued; but often we don't have as much control over that as our inner environment and our reaction to stress. The following remedies can help you to lead a much calmer, energized, and harmonious life in the face of stressful conditions.

- Regular aerobic exercise is a wonderful stress reliever; even nonaerobic exercise such as walking is excellent. Exercise at least three times a week for twenty to thirty minutes a time.

- By far and away, the most effective stress reliever is meditation. Aim for at least one twenty-minute session a day; two or three sessions are even better. You may not feel that you have the time to do this, but if you try it, you might well find that you end up with more energy, and hence, more time. Relaxation techniques are good, too, but I find meditation to be even more beneficial. See Appendix C for a simple meditation technique that I have found quite helpful.

- Flower remedies (solutions containing various flower essences that address different emotional states) are subtle, but very effective over time and they have no side-effects. Ellon USA, Inc. makes English flower remedies according to Dr. Bach's specifications; call their 800 number listed in Appendix A for a catalog and self-help questionnaire. Both English and North American flower remedies can be obtained from Flower Essence Services, whose 800 number is also listed in Appendix A. Call for catalogs and information. In addition, you might be interested in the resources provided by a related nonprofit company, the Flower Essence Society, a referral, networking, and educational service for alternative health care and practitioners. Their toll-free number and Web site is listed in Appendix A as well.

- Several flower essence companies produce and market their own special formula particularly for stress. Bach flowers sells Rescue Remedy and Ellon USA sells Calming Essence.

- BioEnergetics makes a homeopathic stress formula called Stress Release Drops that works quite well. See Appendix A for their 800 number.

- A nice cup of chamomile tea is a soothing treat; the fresher the chamomile, the better.

- Insomnia sufferers may find that taking 5 to 10 mg. of melatonin (available at your local health food store) 30 to 90 minutes before retiring will give them a good night's sleep and not only that, stimulate terrific, vivid dreams. Melatonin is the hormone our pineal gland releases to make us sleepy at night.

  (Incidentally, melatonin is also great for jet lag. Check Appendix B for directions.)

- A pocket diode that helps keep the electromagnetic field of your body in balance is available from The Heritage Store. I wear one in my left pocket and find that when I do, I feel much more relaxed.

- Another technique that can help relieve stress in a big way is to focus in the present as much as possible. A great deal of stress is generated unconsciously by focusing on things in the past that we regret but can't change or worrying about things that might happen in the future. By being fully present in the moment, we get in touch with our own personal source of power much more easily, our intuition and good judgment is sharpened, and we live life more fully. Of course, if your immediate present is rather odious . . . you're in the dentist's chair having your second set of wisdom teeth pulled, for example, or you're trapped at your in-laws watching one of those game shows where everyone screams, loud bells clang, and women who don't know any better actually kiss that guy with the head implant . . . maybe you want to focus on the exhilarating raft trip you experienced last summer or that whale-watching voyage coming up this fall. In general, however, staying focused in the present is a meditative, empowering exercise. Given how we live in this society, you might find it difficult to achieve. Keep at it, though, and you'll find you experience much less stress and depression and much more energy and power.

❖ ❖ ❖

APPENDIX A
Manufacturers and Distributors

BioEnergetics
(800) 334-4043; (503) 668-7478
P O Box 127
Sandy, Oregon 97055
(Allergy drops, Sinus drops, PMS Relief drops, Stress Release drops, among other homeopathic products)

The Grain & Salt Society, Inc.
(800) 867-5800
P O Box 935
Asheville, NC 28815
(Celtic Sea Saltô)

Ellon USA Inc.
(800) 423-2256
644 Merrick Road
Lynbrook, NY 11563
(English flower remedies)

Flower Essence Services
(800) 548-0075, phone
(916) 265-6467, fax
(English and North American flower Remedies)

Flower Essence Society
(800) 736-9222, phone
(916) 265-0584, fax
E-mail address: Info@flowersociety.org
Web site: WWW.flowersociety.org
(Nationwide referral service for alternative health)

Herb Pharm
(800) 348-4372
Williams, OR 97544
(Echinacea)

Home Health
(800) 284-9123
P O Box 2219
Virginia Beach, VA 23450-2219
(Similasan eye drops, and a whole range of health and beauty-related products)

The Heritage Store
(800) 862-2923
P O Box 444-V
Virginia Beach, VA 23458-0444
(Castor oil, Scarmassage, Slim Pocket Diode, powdered vitamin C, Mother Earth Cough Syrup, and other good stuff; the majority of the products are based on remedies provided by Edgar Cayce in his readings)

Shanah Azee (BHI, Heel)
(800) 945-0409, phone
(800) 689-6674, fax
P O Box 26296
Albuquerque, NM 87125-6296
(BHI's Asthma, Arthritis, Cough and Eye tablets, Calendula ointment; Heel's Gripp-Heel tablets, Traumeel ointment and tablets, Euphorbium nasal spray, plus many other homeopathic and herbal remedies).

APPENDIX B
The Natural Medicine Chest

Keep on hand:

Alfalfa tablets (for arthritis, constipation, and flu)
Aloe vera plant (for burns)
Calendula ointment (for burns and hemorrhoids)
Celtic sea salt (for sinus cleanse, sore throat, hot soaks)
Cough tablets
Echinacea (for colds, flu, immune system in general)
Euphorbium nasal spray (for sinus congestion)
Flower remedies (for life's many emotional upsets)
Gripp-Heel (for colds and flu)
Local honey (for allergies and asthma, as well as coughs)
Mother Earth's cough syrup
Scarmassage
Traumeel ointment (for bruises and sprains)
Pocket Diode (for stress, immune system)
Poison Oak/Ivy drops
Psyllium seed and accompanying herb tablets (for constipation)
Similasan eye drops
Sinus drops
Vitamin C (for colds and cold sores)
Vitamin E oil (for fever blister prevention and healing of skin)
Vitamin E capsules (for cramps)
Whiskey (for coughs and colds)
Witch hazel (for insect bites, hemorrhoids)

Optional:

Alum powder (for canker sores)
Arthritis tablets
Allergy drops
Asthma tablets
Astralagus tablets (for immune system)
Boswellin Cream (for arthritis)
Castor oil (for cramps)
Melatonin (for insomnia; also works great for jet lag: Take recommended dosage in section on Stress every night for the number of time zones you have crossed. E.g., if you've crossed 6 time zones, take it for 6 nights, both traveling and when you return.)
Peanut oil (for inflamed joints; also good for low back pain)
PMS Relief drops

APPENDIX C
Meditation Technique

This is a very simple technique, but if practiced over time, it is extremely effective:

Sit in a comfortable, straight-backed chair. You can use a sofa or an armchair, too, if you want, but I find that sometimes I get too comfy and I fall asleep instead of meditating.

Lay your hands in your lap.

Close your eyes.

Breathe regularly and deeply, from your diaphragm or abdomen.

Focus your attention on one of three things: your hands, the center of your forehead, or your hands and the center of your forehead at the same time. I find the combination of focus to be the most effective, but it can be a little tricky. You might want to start out with one or the other. When you focus your attention on either of these areas, you'll feel a slight tingling. Concentrate on that tingling sensation and nothing else.

When mental chatter pipes up or you find yourself becoming distracted by whether or not you left some socks in the dryer or the fact that the person you paid to repair your CD player didn't really repair it but they charged you for it anyway or the fact that squirrels are building a nest in your attic, just become aware of whatever is passing through your mind. Then let it go and return your attention to your hands or the center of your forehead. The longer you can maintain your attention on your focus of meditation, the better. But don't get discouraged if this is very difficult. It takes practice. If you just keep trying, you'll find that little by little, it gets easier and easier.

Do this for twenty minutes, minimum, even if you keep getting distracted. Once a day is good, twice a day is better, and three times a day is ideal.

❖ ❖ ❖

APPENDIX D
How to Take Homeopathic Remedies

Always store homeopathic remedies in a cool, dark, dry place.

When taking homeopathic drops, place them underneath your tongue. Be sure not to touch the dropper on your teeth, lips, or anything else.

When taking homeopathic tablets, dissolve them slowly under your tongue.

Refrain from brushing your teeth, eating, smoking, or drinking anything besides water for fifteen minutes before and after taking a homeopathic remedy.

It's okay to take more than one homeopathic remedy at a time. But if you're taking herbs or vitamins, wait fifteen minutes before taking them. A half hour would be even better.

It would also be helpful to wait fifteen minutes before applying lipstick, mentholated lip balm, scented face creams, perfume, or aftershaves.

Don't store homeopathic tablets in anything besides the container they came in. Don't mix different remedies in the same container.

"Illness and the opportunity it presents people to engage consciously and actively in a journey towards wholeness can be one of the most transformative experiences that life offers."

— *From RITUALS OF HEALING, by J. Achterberg, B. Dossey, and L. Kolkmeier*

About the author

Celeste White, known as "Dr. Bunny" to her friends, has served as a lay healer for common ailments for over ten years. Winner of the Belyea Botany Prize from Wellesley College, where she graduated a Wellesley Scholar, she also possesses a M.S. in Botany from the University of Massachusetts, Amherst, where she studied under a University Fellowship.

If you would like to obtain additional copies of **Natural Remedies for Common Ailments**, check your local health food or book store, or complete and send the order form below, along with your check:

Ship to (please print):

Name _____

Address _____

City, State, Zip _____

Daytime phone _____

_____ copies of **Natural Remedies for Common Ailments** @ $7.95 each

Postage and handling, $2.50 per book _____

California residents add 7.25 % tax _____

Total amount enclosed _____

Make checks payable to
Keswick House

**Send to: Keswick House
P O Box 992535
Redding, CA 96099**